Camila De Paiva Macedo

# Cytotoxicity and Genotoxicity Analysis of Two Endondontic Cements

Camila De Paiva Macedo

# Cytotoxicity and Genotoxicity Analysis of Two Endondontic Cements

## in human fibroblast cultures in vitro

ScienciaScripts

**Imprint**

Any brand names and product names mentioned in this book are subject to trademark, brand or patent protection and are trademarks or registered trademarks of their respective holders. The use of brand names, product names, common names, trade names, product descriptions etc. even without a particular marking in this work is in no way to be construed to mean that such names may be regarded as unrestricted in respect of trademark and brand protection legislation and could thus be used by anyone.

Cover image: www.ingimage.com

This book is a translation from the original published under ISBN 978-613-9-62906-0.

Publisher:
Sciencia Scripts
is a trademark of
Dodo Books Indian Ocean Ltd. and OmniScriptum S.R.L publishing group

120 High Road, East Finchley, London, N2 9ED, United Kingdom
Str. Armeneasca 28/1, office 1, Chisinau MD-2012, Republic of Moldova, Europe
Printed at: see last page
**ISBN: 978-620-7-75671-1**

# SUMMARY

# ACKNOWLEDGMENTS

First of all, thank God for the gift of life. You have supported me on this journey, without your presence nothing could have happened.

To my beloved parents Helena and Nelson, who have always been and always will be by my side, giving me the strength to always strive for the best, without whom this dream would never come true. To my sister Marina who is the light of my life, always believing and encouraging me every day of my journey. To my grandmother Lélia and my aunt Heloisa, who have supported me through the most difficult times.

To all my family in Americana-SP (Aunt Leà, Uncle José Maria, Andréa and Léo) who welcomed me with immense love and affection, without whom I would not have been able to complete this stage. To my beloved nieces Fernanda and Carol, who taught me the purest form of love.

To my esteemed advisor Prof. Dr. Alexandre Sigrist De Martin for passing on his knowledge, for his dedication and attention to me and especially for his immense patience in teaching me. Thank you very much!

To the coordinator of the Master's program, Prof. Dr. Carlos Eduardo da Silveira Bueno, for the honor of knowing him and being his student, never sparing any effort in passing on his knowledge.

To Prof. Dr. Sérgio Luiz Pinheiro for his immense contribution in the execution of this work, his collaboration was extremely important in the preparation of this Dissertation.

Thanks to Prof. Dr. Elizabeth Martinez and biologist Polyanna Montaldi for their availability, guidance and help in carrying out the laboratory part of this research.

To the Sao Leopoldo Mandic Dental Research Center, for the excellence of the course and all the structure offered.

To the teaching staff of the Campinas Endodontics Team, who contributed greatly to my professional and personal learning.

To my great friend and encourager Eduardo Marques, thank you for your trust and for all the knowledge you've passed on over the years.

Finally, to my very special friends that the Master's gave me. Thank you for all your support, encouragement and immense affection. Thank you for making me grow professionally. I've learned a lot from all these friends, they're all forever in my life.

# SUMMARY

The aim of this *in vitro* study was to evaluate the cytotoxic and genotoxic potential of MTA Fillapex endodontic cement compared to AH plus cement. Human fibroblast cell lines FG11 and FG15 were used for this study. Cytotoxicity and genotoxicity were analyzed in human gingival fibroblasts subjected to conditioned cell culture medium by MTT reduction assay and micronucleus formation test respectively. Cells cultured in DMEM medium served as a control. Cell viability was measured at 24, 48 and 72 hours. The results were analyzed using Biostat 4.0. The Shapiro Wilk normality test was performed and the sample showed non-normal behavior. A descriptive analysis was carried out and the results were submitted to the Kruskal-Wallis (Dunn) test. All the cements and the control group showed lower MTT values at 24 hours compared to 48 and 72 hours (p<00001). Higher cell viability was observed in AH Plus cement and the control group compared to MTA Fillapex in all experimental periods (p<0.0001). In relation to genotoxicity, the highest value was observed in AH Plus cement in the 24-hour period, with a significant difference in relation to MTA Fillapex and the control group (p=0.0004). It can be concluded that MTA Fillapex cement showed greater cellular cytotoxicity than the two groups and in the genotoxicity test, AH Plus cement showed greater gentoxicity than the other groups.

**Keywords:** Cytotoxicity, Genotoxicity, Fibroblasts.

# DISSEMINATION AND TRANSFER OF KNOWLEDGE

Once the root canal system has been properly instrumented and disinfected, the canal space should be filled with cements that damage the tissues around the root canal as little as possible. For this reason, a cement must be used to ensure that the root canal system is properly sealed, thus preventing the entry of oral fluids, as it is known that contact with bacteria, chemicals and tissue remains can generate inflammatory responses in the body, impairing the recovery of the tissues adjacent to the root canal. The aim of this study was to show that two cements used in root canal treatment can cause damage to the body's cells and genetic material. Biocompatibility tests called the cytotoxicity test and the genotoxicity test were carried out. The results observed here showed that one cement caused greater damage to the cells and the other cement caused greater damage to the cells' genetic material.

# 1. INTRODUCTION

After correct instrumentation and adequate disinfection, the root canal space must be filled with biocompatible materials (Nguyen, 1987; Taintor et al., 1978). The characteristics and physico-chemical properties of endodontic cements are fundamental to achieving a good seal, and an adequate coronal restoration tends to prevent bacterial micro-infiltration (Ray & Trope., 1995; Santos et al., 2010).

This sealing promoted by the cements used to fill the root canal system aims to prevent the entry of oral fluids along the canal, including irregularities of the apical foramen and slight discrepancies of the root canal dentin wall with the filling material (Branstetter & Von Fraunhofer., 1982), reducing the possibility of recontamination of the prepared space (Walton & Torabinejad., 2002).

Some types of endodontic cements are available on the market. In particular, bioceramic-based materials, which generally contain calcium silicate and/or calcium phosphate, have attracted attention due to their physical and biological properties, such as alkaline pH, chemical stability in biological tissues and lack of shrinkage. They are also considered non-toxic and biocompatible (Candeiro et al., 2012; Loushine et al., 2011; Zhang et al., 2009).

The trend is for more and more cements to have characteristics such as: good tissue tolerance, the ability to be resorbed at the peri-apex in the event of leakage, stimulating or allowing the deposition of mineralized tissue in the apex region, being easy to insert, being plastic at the time of insertion and becoming solid afterwards, have a good working time, provide a good seal, not shrink, not be permeable, have good viscosity and adherence, not be soluble inside the root canal, have a pH close to neutral, thus combining physical, chemical and biological properties (Leonardo et al., 2008).

Biocompatibility and sealing capacity are extremely important characteristics and various endodontic cements have been developed with the aim of improving these features (Schilder, 1967; Scarparo et al., 2009; Scarparo et al., 2010; Nagas et al., 2012).

Many parameters characterize the biocompatibility of a material, such as cytotoxicity, genotoxicity, mutagenicity and carcinogenicity (Al-Hiyasat et al., 2010). The presence of a toxic effect *in vitro* does not mean that the material is toxic when applied *in vivo*. On the other hand, the absence of a toxic effect *in vitro* is possibly a guarantee of a good clinical response. In addition, the *in vitro* test provides guidance as to the duration and intensity of cytotoxic and genotoxic effects, and may even indicate against the clinical use of a material if it falls outside a minimum standard of toxicity (Senne et al., 2009).

The MTT 3-(4,5 dimethylthiazol-2yl)-2,5-diphenyl-tetrazolium assay has been widely used as a cytotoxicity test in cell cultures. The method for assessing cytotoxicity using the MTT dye has proved to be extremely reliable, fast and easily reproducible, reflecting not only the number of cells in a sample, but also the level of their metabolic activity, as it is based on the activity of enzymes present in viable cells (Bouillaguet et al., 2004).

Kim et al. (2007) studied the effectiveness of the MTT test for verifying the viability of periodontal ligament cells. For these authors, MTT is a fast, highly effective test that is easy to manipulate and immediately provides the quantity and identification of viable cells. Similarly, Eldeniz et al. (2007) agree with the effectiveness of contacting cells with different products and consider this test to be simple, quick and with results that are close to reality.

Genotoxicity tests can be defined as *in vitro* and *in vivo* tests and are designed to detect components that induce damage to the genetic material of cells such as DNA breakage, genetic mutation, chromosomal breakage and alteration in DNA repair capacity (Ribeiro et al., 2006). In recent decades, genotoxicity tests have been widely accepted as an important carcinogenic indicator. *In vitro* genotoxicity tests include the comet test and the micronucleus test (Ribeiro et al., 2004).

Currently, resin cements are more prominent in the endodontic clinic, but despite their great popularity, they are capable of promoting cytotoxicity and mutagenicity (Schweikl et al., 2000, Huang et al., 2002).

MTA Fillapex (Angelus, Londrina, PR, Brazil), a cement based on calcium silicate, was recently introduced to the market. Its composition after manipulation is basically MTA, natural resin, bismuth oxide and silica nanoparticles. According to the manufacturer, it has excellent radiopacity, easy handling, a long working time and low solubility, providing a seal by expanding when it sets.

Gomes-Filho et al. (2012) described a similar tissue response when compared to the original MTA formulation, and the biological responses of MTA Fillapex compared to other endodontic cements.

AH Plus (Dentsply/De Trey, Konstanz, Germany) is an epoxyamine resin-based cement. It consists of 2 pastes, A and B, whose main components are calcium tungstateate, zirconium oxide, iron oxide, amine adamantate, silicone oil and others (Lopes and Siqueira, 2010). This cement has good apical sealing capacity and excellent histological behavior, allowing biological sealing through the deposition of cementoid tissue (Leonardo et al., 1999). It also has satisfactory antibacterial activity and good drainage (Siqueira et al., 2000). For Cohen et al. (2011) one of the main characteristics of AH Plus cement is that it offers adhesion and does not contain eugenol.

Contact with microbial, mechanical and chemical irritants, either alone or in combination, can generate periapical inflammatory responses of varying intensities, depending on the degree of aggression, which can impair the tissue repair process. Therefore, the evaluation of the irritant potential of new products appearing on the market is generally carried out on animals, prior to testing on human beings. Recently, several alternative *in vitro* methods for testing the toxic potential of some materials have been proposed *in* preference to *in vivo* tests (Lee et al., 2000).

Given the range of products available for endodontic treatment, especially the resin endodontic cements used to fill root canals, it is of great importance to study the effects that these materials can have on the tissues adjacent to the periapical region. The purpose of this study was to evaluate the cytotoxic and genotoxic potential of two resin endodontic cements used to fill root canal systems *in vitro*.

# 2.  LITERATURE REVIEW

Schmalz (1994) mentions that the study of biocompatibility is extremely important, since endodontic materials of the most different types and compositions remain in direct or indirect contact with apical and periapical tissues for an indefinite period of time. The toxicity of a dental material can be assessed by *in vitro* tests, animal experiments or *in vivo* clinical studies. *In vitro* tests are the most widely used to assess the cytotoxicity or genotoxicity of a material used in dentistry. For dental materials, the cell culture technique is the most suitable and widely used; contact between the cells and the materials to be tested can occur directly or indirectly.

Torabinejad et al. (1995) carried out a study on the cytotoxicity of four retrofilling materials: amalgam, Super EBA, IRM and MTA using a cell culture method (L929 rat fibroblasts), the authors observed that the material which showed the lowest degree of cytotoxicity was MTA followed by amalgam, Super EBA and IRM.They could conclude that MTA is a very satisfactory retrograde obturator material from a chemical-physical-biological point of view, especially because of its biocompatibility and its potential for osteoconductive action.

Schweikl & Schmalz. (2000) checked the cytotoxicity and genotoxicity of AH Plus cement and its components (paste A and paste B) by means of micronucleus induction in V79 cells. AH Plus was tested immediately after handling and after 24 hours. Pastes A and B diluted in DMSO reduced the viability of V79 cells, and the number of micronuclei was seven times higher in treated cell cultures compared to the untreated control.

After 24 hours, no genotoxicity was observed in AH Plus diluted with DMSO or physiological saline. However, the authors showed that AH Plus induced chromosomal mutations immediately after manipulation.

Huang et al. (2002) evaluated the cytotoxicity of different resin-based endodontic cements (AH 26, AH Plus), those based on zinc oxide and eugenol (Canals, Endomethasone and N2) and those based on calcium hydroxide (Sealapex) on human periodontal ligament cells and V79 hamster cells. The results showed that all the cements were cytotoxic to both cell cultures, with calcium hydroxide-based cement being the least toxic of the others tested.

Miletic et al. (2003) compared AH 26 and AH Plus in terms of cytotoxicity and genotoxicity in V79 cells. To analyze cytotoxicity, the extracts of the cements were prepared in dilutions of DMSO and the cultures were stained with Nigrosin dye at 1h, 24h and 7 days. The genotoxicity of the cements was assessed by the formation of micronuclei in human lymphocytes. Both cements showed similar cytotoxicity at high concentrations; however, they did not induce chromosomal aberrations or the formation of abnormal micronuclei in any experimental period.

In 2005, Miletic et al. evaluated the cytotoxicity of RoekoSeal Automix (RSA) and AH Plus cement on L929 rat fibroblast cells and human cervical carcinoma cells (HeLa) at 1h, 24h, 48h, 7 days and 1 month. The results showed that AH Plus was significantly more toxic at 1h, 24h and 48h compared to 7 days and 1 month in both cell lines. RoekoSeal, on the other hand, had no cytotoxic effect on both cell lines and in all evaluation periods.

Kim et al. (2007) studied the effectiveness of the 3-(4,5 dimethylthiazol-2yl)-2,5-diphenyl-tetrazolium bromide (MTT) dye method for checking the viability of periodontal ligament cells. MTT has been used for cytotoxicity tests on cell cultures, assessing their mitochondrial metabolism. For these authors, it is a quick test, highly effective, easy to manipulate and immediately provides the quantity and identification of viable cells. Similarly, Eldeniz et al (2007) agree with the effectiveness of MTT in assessing cell metabolism after contact between cells and different products and consider this test to be simple, quick and guarantee real results.

Lodiene et al. (2008) compared the toxicity of AH Plus, EndoREZ, RoekoSeal and Epiphany using the filter diffusion and MTT tests on L929 fibroblasts. The cement specimens were prepared in 5mm diameter non-reactive plastic rings and used by direct contact in the Millipore filter diffusion test and in the form of extracts (indirect contact) in the MTT test.The filter diffusion test showed that Epiphany and AH Plus, when placed in contact with the cells immediately after handling the cements (setting time 0h), were severely toxic, while RoekoSeal and EndoREZ were non-toxic. When they reached a hardening time of 24 hours, Epiphany showed moderate toxicity, while AH Plus, RoekoSeal and EndoREZ showed no toxicity. In the MTT test when hardened, Epiphany proved to be severely more toxic than the other materials.

Leonardo et al. (2008) evaluated the biocompatibility of RoekoSeal cement with the periapical tissues of dogs and compared it with AH Plus. The pulps of 32 teeth were removed, the apical cementum was perforated, biomechanical preparation was carried out and the canals were filled using the lateral condensation technique. Ninety days after surgery, the animals were euthanized, the tooth and bone block was removed and the samples were prepared for microscopic analysis. In the RoekoSeal group, mineralized tissue was deposited, with complete neoformation of apical tissue in 43.8% of the teeth and partial sealing in 56.2%. In the AH Plus group, 12.5% had complete neoformation of mineralized apical tissue, 75% had partial sealing and 12.5% had no sealing. There was no difference between the groups in terms of inflammatory infiltrate, periodontal ligament thickness and resorption of dentin, cementum or bone. RoekoSeal showed satisfactory biological responses when compared to the effects of AH Plus.

Scarparo et al. (2009) investigated the reaction of subcutaneous connective tissue in rats. Polyethylene tubes filled with the cements were implanted in 18 rats and they were grouped according to three experimental periods (7, 30 and 60 days). Inflammatory reactions were assessed in four groups: Group I methacrylate-based cement (EndoREZ; Ultradent, Inc, South Jordan, UT), Group II epoxy resin-based cement (AH Plus, Dentsply D Trey, GmbH Konstanz, Germany), Group III zinc oxide and eugenol-based cement (Endofill, Dentsply Industria e Comercio Ltda, Petrópolis, RJ, Brazil) and Group IV, the control group (empty tube). The authors observed that the samples containing EndoREZ and Endofill cements showed more intense and long-lasting inflammation, while the sample with AH Plus showed a decrease in inflammatory reaction over time and in the control group there was a reduction in inflammatory cells. None of the cements tested exhibited ideal biocompatibility characteristics.

Senne et al. (2009) evaluated the cytotoxicity of two epoxy resin-based cements (Sealer 26 and AH Plus) and a zinc oxide and eugenol-based cement (Endofill) on the VERO C1008 cell line. Cytotoxicity was assessed using the FluoroQuenchTM AO/EB reagent, and the use of LB Rapid Panothic dye (Laborclin), a differentiated staining system widely used in hematology, was used to assess morphological changes in the cells, immediately after manipulation with the fresh cement and 24, 48 and 72 hours after contact with the cements. The cements were manipulated according to the manufacturer's recommendations for the experiment with hardened cements, which were stored for one night, about 12h, in ultraviolet light, in order to prevent any contamination before coming into contact with the cell suspension. All the plates were incubated at 37°C and observations were made at 24, 48 and 72 hours. After 12 hours, 2µl of cell suspension at a concentration of $3.5 \times 10^5$ was poured over the cements. After 1 hour, 5µl of FluoroQuenchTM dye was poured into each well. Observation was made of the relative extent corresponding to the areas of fluorecenste green staining, representative of viable cells, in each sample exposed to the cements. The measurement was carried out using Imagem Pro Plus software (Media Cybernetic) and submitted to the Student's t-test. They concluded that all the cements tested were cytotoxic at some point, showing different levels of proliferation and cell morphology. Endofill cement, based on zinc oxide and eugenol, was highly cytotoxic both fresh and after hardening. Sealer 26 behaved in a similar way, but at 24 hours it was significantly better than Endofill when hardened. AH Plus was the cement that showed the best results in terms of the morphological aspect of the cells after hardening and the lowest cytotoxicity.

Al-Hiyasat et al. (2010) evaluated the cytotoxicity of four endodontic cements, AH Plus, EndoREZ, Epiphany and MetaSeal on C 3T3 fibroblast cells. The cements were handled according to the manufacturer's recommendations. One gram of each material was placed in the bottom of 6-well plates in the form of approximately 20 disks weighing approximately 50 grams each. The specimens were covered with 10mL of PBS and left for a week in an oven at 37° C and 5% $CO_2$. After this period, 10µl of the original extracts and a dilution of 1 in 10v/v were placed in contact with 90µl of cell culture for 48 hours at 37° C and 5% $CO_2$; the control group was treated with the same amount of PBS. Cytotoxic activity was assessed using the MTT test. In the original extracts, all the materials reduced viability, AH Plus showed the least cytotoxicity, followed by EndoRez, Epiphany and MetaSeal. In the dilution of the original extract, AH Plus was less cytotoxic, followed by Epiphany, EndoRez and MetaSeal. The dilution of the original extract reduced the viability of MetaSeal from 11% to 9.5%.

According to Soares and Goldberg (2011), zinc oxide and eugenol-based cements (such as Endofill and Fillcanal) are widely used. However, despite having good physicochemical properties, they do not behave favorably in terms of biocompatibility. Their action on the subcutaneous tissues of rats revealed the presence of a chronic inflammatory process, leading to tissue damage, attributed to the presence of free eugenol which can remain for prolonged periods of time, acting as a cell depressant.

In 2011, Karapinar-Kazandag et al. studied the cytotoxicity of AH Plus, EndoREZ, RoekoSeal, Epiphany and Activ GP on L929 fibroblasts and primary human pulp cells using the MTS test. The specimens were prepared, placed in Teflon rings (4 mm diameter/2 mm height), kept in an oven until the hardening period provided by the manufacturer and placed in 2.5 mL of culture medium for 1, 4 and 7 days in an oven at 37°C. The original extracts and two dilutions (25% and 50%) were used for the tests. Activ GP and Epiphany cements were significantly more toxic than the other cements, but their cytotoxicity decreased when the extracts were diluted. Epiphany became more toxic after 7 days. No or minimal toxicity was observed with RoekoSeal, AH Plus and EndoREZ.

Bin et al. (2012) carried out a study comparing the cytotoxicity and genotoxicity of MTA Fillapex cement to AH Plus cement and white MTA. Chinese hamster fibroblast cells (V79) were previously placed in contact with different dilutions of culture. Cytotoxicity was assessed using the metol-thiazole-diphenyl tetrazolium spectrophotometer assay to check cell viability and survival rates. Genotoxicity was assessed using the micronucleus formation assay. The cell survival rate and the number of micronuclei were evaluated before and after exposure to the endodontic cements and the results were statistically analyzed. In this study, the results showed that cell viability remained above 50% in the white MTA group at all dilutions. Both AH Plus and MTA Fillapex showed the lowest rates of cell viability and caused an increase in the formation of micronuclei when compared to the control group. The authors show in this study that MTA Fillapex showed the highest cytotoxicity, while white MTA was considered the least toxic and genotoxic in contact with Chinese hamster fibroblast cell culture (V79).

Gomes-Filho et al. (2012) evaluated the reaction of the subcutaneous tissue of rats to the implantation of polyethylene tubes filled with MTA Fillapex compared to the reaction to tubes filled with Sealapex and white MTA. In this study, MTA Fillapex caused a moderate inflammatory response at 7 days, which was reduced over time, similar to white MTA. In addition, Sealapex, white MTA and MTA Fillapex stimulated the formation of mineralized tissue. The authors concluded that MTA Fillapex is a biocompatible material.

Yoshino et al. (2013) compared the cytotoxicity of white MTA, MTA Fillapex and Portland cement on human periodontal ligament fibroblasts. A culture of periodontal ligament fibroblasts was established and the cells were used for cytotoxic tests after four passages. Cell density was adjusted to $1.24 \times 10^4$ in 96-well plates. Extracts of endodontic material were prepared and inserted into specimens (5x3mm) in 1 mL of culture medium for 72h. The extracts were diluted twice and inserted into the wells and seeded by cells for 24h, 48h and 72h. The MTT assay was used to analyze cell viability. White MTA showed a cytotoxic effect in the 24h and 72h extracts, while Fillapex MTA showed the highest cytotoxic levels with reduced cell viability in pure and diluted extracts. In this study, Portland cement showed no changes in the cell viability of fibroblasts. They concluded that MTA Fillapex was the material that showed the greatest cytotoxic effect on human periodontal ligament fibroblasts, followed by white MTA and Portland cement.

Marques et al. (2013) carried out a study to evaluate the response of rat subcutaneous tissue to MTA Fillapex, experimental endodontic cement based on Portland cement with added propylene glycol and paste containing zinc oxide and eugenol with iodoform. At 7 days, the inflammatory response was intense in the zinc oxide and eugenol paste with iodoform group. During this period, the MTA Fillapex group showed some giant cells, macrophages and lymphocytes. At 15 days, the MTA Fillapex group showed the presence of fibroblasts and collagen fibers, indicating a process of tissue healing. Portland cement showed similar results to MTA Fillapex. The zinc oxide and eugenol cement with iodoform group showed less favorable biological behavior, with intense infiltration, even after 15 days. The authors concluded that MTA Fillapex and Portland cement are more biocompatible.

Silva et al. (2013) tested the cytotoxicity and pH of MTA Fillapex and AH Plus. The pH level was measured at intervals of 3h, 24h, 72h and 168h. The authors found that MTA Fillapex was more cytotoxic than AH Plus in all four-week periods, when testing the viability of mouse fibroblasts (Balb/c 3T3), maintaining constant cytotoxicity over time. AH Plus was moderately cytotoxic initially, slightly cytotoxic after one week and became non-cytotoxic after two weeks. Regarding the pH results of the cements tested, the authors observed that MTA Fillapex showed an alkaline pH at all experimental times, while AH Plus showed a neutral pH value.

Gomes-Filho et al. (2013) carried out a study to assess the repair of periapical lesions in canine teeth after single-session endodontic treatment and obturation with MTA Fillapex, Sealapex and Endo- CPM-Sealer. The results obtained were unsatisfactory, regardless of the cement used. These findings showed that the cements used were unable to combat the endodontic infection remaining after the canal repair was completed, as the periapical tissues were not completely repaired. It should be noted that in teeth filled with MTA Fillapex and Sealapex, the inflammatory reaction in the periapical region, in close contact with the materials, was less intense, demonstrating better biocompatibility. The study showed that even with the use of biocompatible materials that stimulate mineralization, repair does not occur without disinfecting the root canal system.

Couto et al. (2014) carried out a study to analyze the cytotoxicity of MTA Fillapex in *vitro* using gingival fibroblasts cultured in *Dulbecco's modified Eagle Medium* (DMEM) and submitted to culture medium conditioned with MTA or MTA Fillapex. This conditioned medium contained substances released by endodontic cements. Cells cultured in fresh medium served as a positive control. Cell viability was assessed by MTT assay after 1, 3, 5 and 7 days. The authors obtained the following results: The cells submitted to the MTA-conditioned medium showed a cell growth curve similar to that of the cells in the control group, for the MTA Fillapex group, there was no cell growth and a significantly lower number of viable cells was observed than in the other groups during the experiment. Thus, the authors concluded that the substances released from MTA Fillapex did not allow cell growth, showing that this MTA-based endodontic cement is highly cytotoxic. The biocompatibility characteristics of MTA may be lost with MTA Fillapex and compromise the success of endodontic treatment.

Also in 2014, Chang et al. carried out a study in which the aim was to compare the cytotoxicity of four endodontic cements: Sealapex (Sybron Kerr, WA), Apatite root sealer (ARS; Dentsply Sankin, Tokyo, Japan), MTA Fillapex (Angellus Industria de Produtos Odontológicos S/A, Londrina, PR, Brazil) and iRoot SP (Innovate BioCreamix Inc, Vancouver, Canada) on human periodontal ligament cells. Cytotoxicity was assessed using 3-(4,5 dimethylthiazolyl-2yl)- 2,5 diphenyltetrazolium bromide assays. The cements were handled according to the manufacturers and were placed in disks with a diameter of 6 mm and a height of 2 mm. The samples were conditioned at $37^0$ C in 100% humidity to allow them to set. All the samples were sterilized using gamma radiation. After exposing the materials for 3, 7 and 14 days, viable cells were detected. Cell viability was determined using the MTT assay. The MTT results revealed that none of the cements evaluated had cytotoxic effects. MTA Fillapex showed favorable growth compared to Sealapex, ARS and iRoot SP for 14 days.

Zhou et al. (2015) carried out a study to evaluate the cytotoxicity of 2 endodontic cements containing calcium silicate. The cements were tested using human gingival fibroblasts. The cements evaluated were EndoSequence BC, MTA Fillapex and the control cement was AH Plus. The human gingival fibroblasts were incubated for 3 days with the fresh specimens in DMEM (Dulbecco's modified) culture medium. Human gingival fibroblasts cultured in DMEM medium were used as a control group. Cytotoxicity was assessed by flow cytometry analysis and cell viability at various concentrations (1:2, 1:8, 1:32 and 1:128). In this study, the authors observed that MTA Fillapex was more toxic than AH plus and BC Sealer at concentrations of 1:2 and 1:8. At concentrations of 1:32 and 1:128, MTA Fillapex was not cytotoxic. The authors concluded that BC Sealer and MTA Fillapex (cements containing calcium silicate in their composition) have different cytotoxicity for human gingival fibroblasts.

Silva et al. (2016) conducted a study to evaluate the cytotoxic effects of five endodontic cements (AH Plus, Endomethasone E, EndoSequence BC, MTA Fillapex and Pulp Canal Sealer EWT) using a three-dimensional (3D) cell culture model. A conventional two-dimensional (2D) cell culture model was used as a reference technique for comparison. Balb/c 3T3 fibroblasts were grown in standard two-dimensional cell culture and the three-dimensional cell culture models in type I rat tail collagen. Both cell cultures were then incubated with the manipulated endodontic cements for 24 hours. Cell viability was measured using the MTT assay. All the cements tested exhibited cytotoxic effects. MTA Fillapex was much more cytotoxic than the other endodontic cements tested. Thus, the authors concluded that cytotoxicity was greater in two-dimensional cell cultures than in three-dimensional cell cultures. EndoSequence BC cement exhibited greater biocompatibility and MTA Fillapex cement less biocompatibility.

# 3.  PROPOSAL

The aim of this *in vitro* study was to analyze and compare the cytotoxic and genotoxic potential of two endodontic cements: MTA Fillapex and AH Plus in human fibroblast cultures.

The null hypothesis is that both cements show the same behavior in the two tests.

# 4. MATERIALS AND METHODS

## 4.1 Materials

Table 1 - Materials with their respective manufacturers, brands, city and country.

| MATERIALS | MANUFACTURER / CITY / COUNTRY |
| --- | --- |
| AH Plus | Dentsply, Konstanz, Germany |
| Trypan blue | Sigm-Aldrich, (Corporation, Detroit, USA) |
| Neubauer-Fisher camera | Scientific (Pittisburgh, USA) |
| Laminar flow hood | Veco Flow Ltda, (Campinas-Brazil) |
| Greenhouse | Thermo Scientific Farma Series II (Savannah, USA) |
| ELX800 multi-plate reader | Epoch Biotek instruments, Chicago, USA |
| Human fibroblast cell lines | Cell Bank of the Cellular and Molecular Biology Laboratory of the Sâo Leopoldo Mandic College (Campinas-Brazil) |
| Dulbecco's Modified Essential Medium (DMEM) | Nutricell (Campinas-Brazil) |
| Inverted phase microscope | Nikon, Eclipse TS 100, Detroit, USA |
| Fluorescence microscope | Carl Zeiss, Oberkochen, Germany |
| MTA Fillapex | Angelus, Londrina-Brazil |
| 24-well thermometer well plate | Econolab Produtos para Laboratòrio Ltda (São Paulo, Brazil) |
| 96-well thermometer well plate | Econolab Produtos para Laboratòrio Ltda (São Paulo, Brazil) |
| Antimycotic antibiotic solution | Sigma, St. Louis, Missouri, USA |
| Formaldehyde solution | Cultilab (Campinas-Brazil) |
| Hoeschst solution | Sigma, St. Louis, Missouri, USA |
| 100% methanol solution | Cultilab (Campinas-Brazil) |

| 10% sodium dodecyl sulfate (SDS) solution | Cultilab (Campinas-Brazil) |
| --- | --- |
| PBS saline solution | Cultilab (Campinas-Brazil) |
| Bovine fetal serum | Cultilab (Campinas-Brazil) |
| Trypsin | Nutricell (Campinas-Brazil) |

## 4.2 Methodology

This study was approved by the Research Ethics Committee of the Sao Leopoldo Mandic School in Campinas, under CEP protocol: 63345516.0.0000.5374 (ANNEX A).

The research was carried out at the Faculty of Dentistry of the Sao Leopoldo Mandic Research Center, Campinas campus, Cellular and Molecular Biology laboratory.

This study used human fibroblast cell lines FG11 and FG15 from the cell bank of the Cellular and Molecular Biology laboratory at the Sao Leopoldo Mandic School (ANNEX B). The cytotoxicity of the sealing cements used in endodontic therapy was assessed 24, 48 and 72 hours after incubation, cell proliferation was assessed using the Trypan blue vital exclusion method and cell viability was assessed using the MTT method in gingival fibroblasts. The number of 4 repetitions per group was obtained from the sample calculation made after the pilot procedure. The ANOVA statistical test was used for the sample calculation, with a minimum difference between the means of the treatments of 0.02, number of treatments of 3, power of the test of 0.80 and alpha of 0.05. The number of replications required was 4.

The AH Plus and MTA Fillapex cements (figure 1) were handled at room temperature (approximately 25°C). According to the manufacturer's instructions, equal quantities (1:1) of paste A and paste B were mixed on a glass plate using a metal spatula. Each sample was inserted into silicone devices 6 mm in diameter and 2 mm high (figure 2), allowing them to set in 24 hours at 37°C in an environment with 100% humidity. They were dried for 24 hours at room temperature and sterilized by 37.2 Gy gamma radiation before being added to the cell culture.

Figure 1- AH Plus and MTA Fillapex cements.

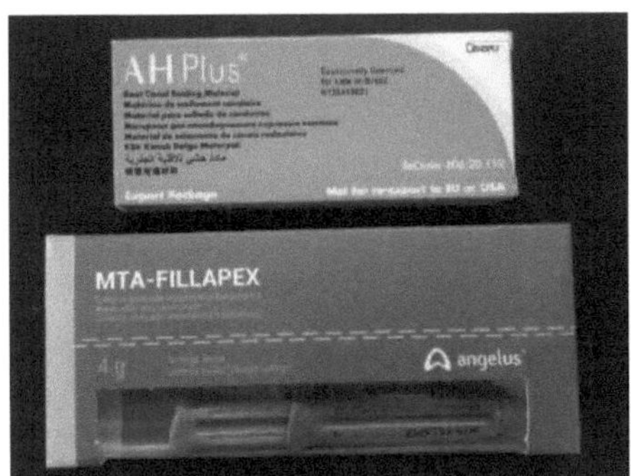

Source: Author

Figura 2-        Specimens inserted into the silicone device.

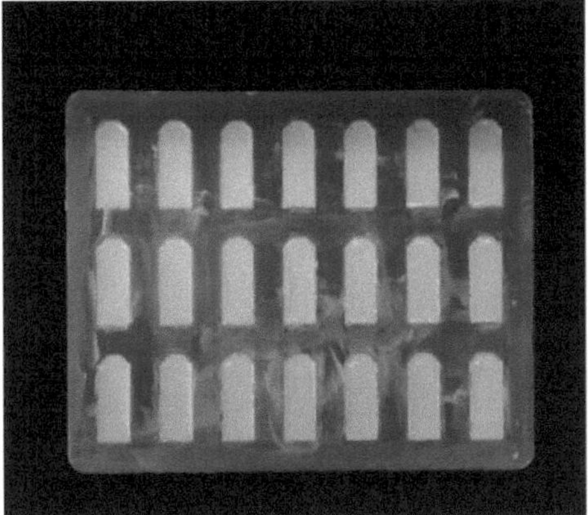

Source: Own authorship.

For this study, the tested cements were divided into experimental groups, with 4 samples for each group, as follows:

(1)  control, DMEM culture;

(2)  DMEM solution containing MTA Fillapex cement;

(3)  DMEM solution containing AH Plus cement;

### 3.2.1 Cell Lineage

To evaluate the cytotoxicity of apical sealing cements used in endodontic therapy in human fibroblast cultures, two strains (FG11 and FG15) obtained from the cell bank of the Cellular and Molecular Biology laboratory at the Sao Leopoldo Mandic School were used. These cells were previously isolated by primary cultivation of human gums removed from three different patients using the explant technique.

### 3.2.2 Cell Cultivation

The fibroblast cells were cultured in Dulbecco's Modified Essential Minimal Medium (DMEM) (Nutricell®, Campinas, SP, Brazil) supplemented with 10% fetal bovine serum (Cultilab®, Campinas, SP, Brazil) and 1% antibiotic-antimycotic solution (Sigma, St. Louis, Missouri, USA).

All procedures were carried out in a laminar flow hood to maintain the sterility of the materials and substances used for cell cultivation.

The fibroblast cells were kept in a greenhouse at 37°C in a humid atmosphere. The culture medium was changed every 2-3 days and the progress of the culture was assessed using an inverted phase microscope.

Figura 3- Dulbeco Modified Essential Medium (DMEM)

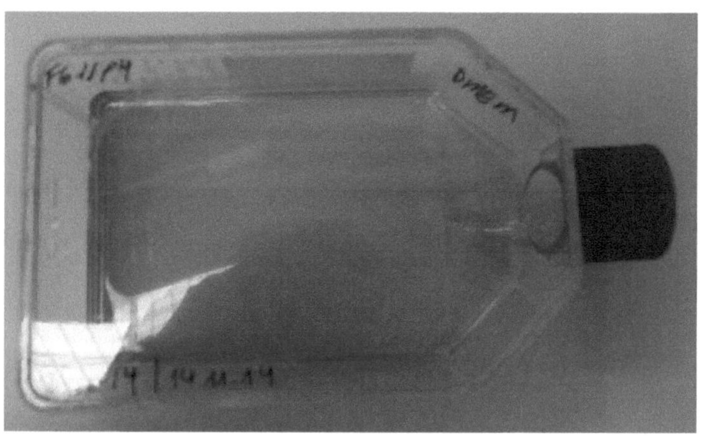

Source: Own authorship.

Figure 4 Greenhouse at 37°C in a humid atmosphere.

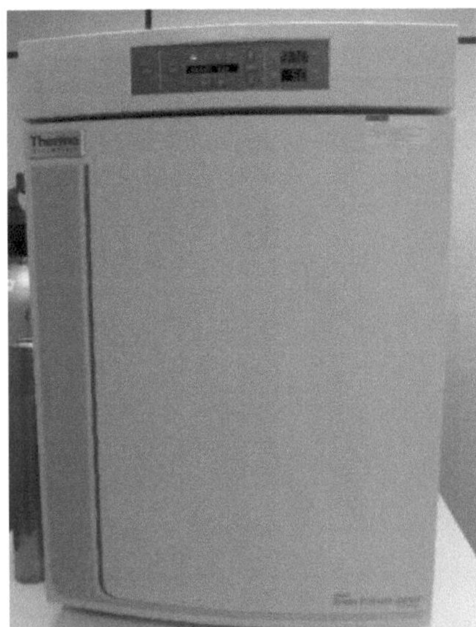

Source: Own authorship.

### 4.2.3 Cell proliferation

The cell suspension was obtained by trypsinizing the 24-well thermometer wells (figure 5) with trypsin (figure 6), which was then inactivated with the culture medium itself and evaluated in a Neubauer chamber under an inverted phase microscope.

To assess cell proliferation, the Trypan blue vital exclusion method was used (figure 7) at 24-hour, 48-hour and 72-hour intervals for each cement tested.

Figure 5- 24-well thermometer plate.

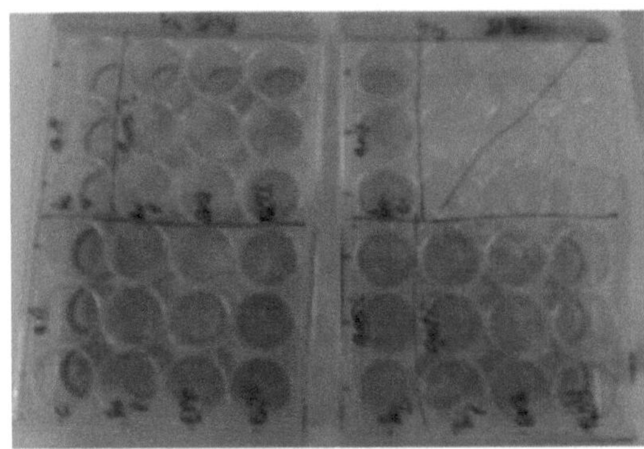

Source: Own authorship.

Figure 6- Trypsin

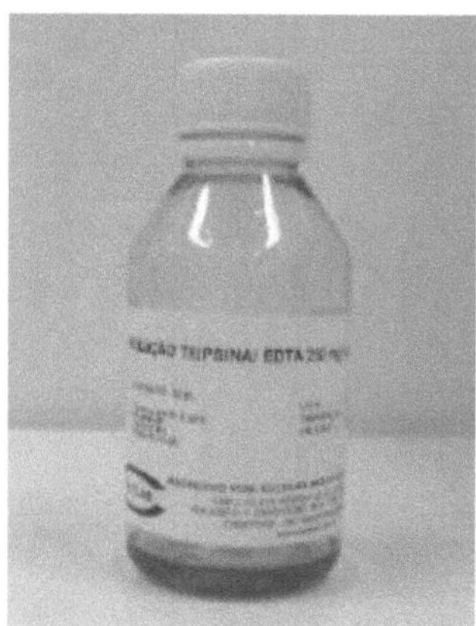

Source: Own authorship.

Figure 7- Trypan blue

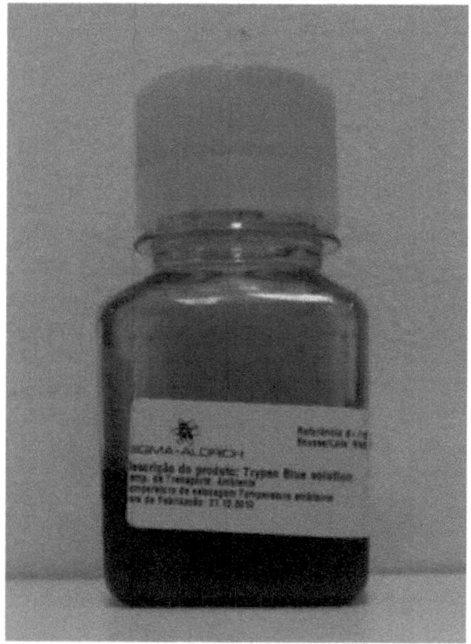

Source: Own authorship.

To do this, after reaching subconfluence, the cells were enzymatically removed from the plates and the precipitate of cells resulting from the centrifugation was suspended in 1 mL of medium (figure 8). 10 µL of the cell suspension was removed (figure 9) and 10 µL of Trypan blue was added to it, and 1 µL of this solution was placed in a hemocytometer (Neubauer chamber - Fisher Scientific, Pittsburgh, PA, USA) (figure 10) and taken to the inverted phase microscope to count and observe the cells.

Figure 8- Eppendorf centrifuge

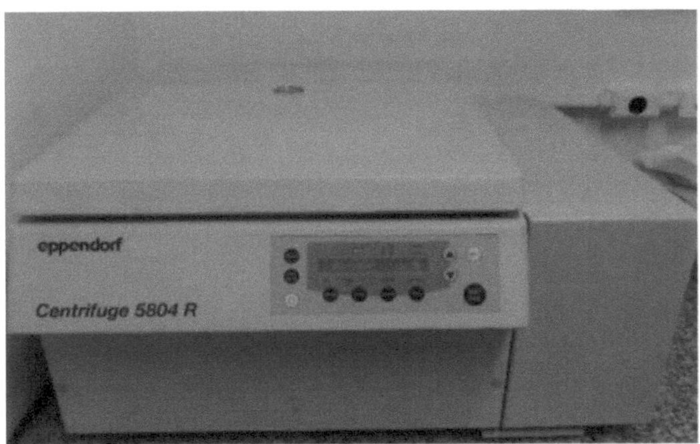


Source: Own authorship.

Figure 9- Neubauer-Fisher camera

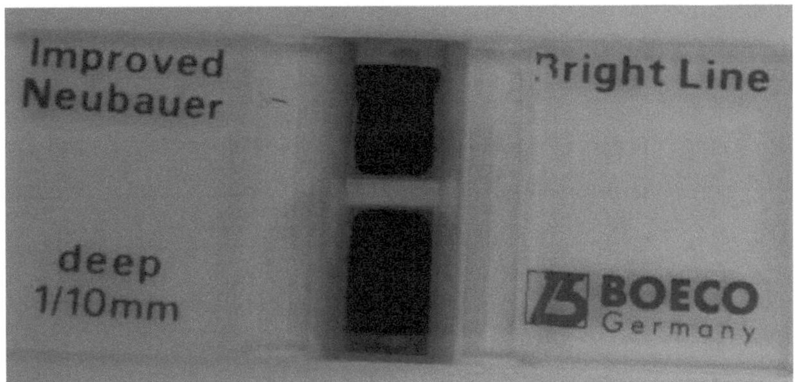


Source: Own authorship.

Figure 10- Cell Counting in the Neubauer-Fisher Camera

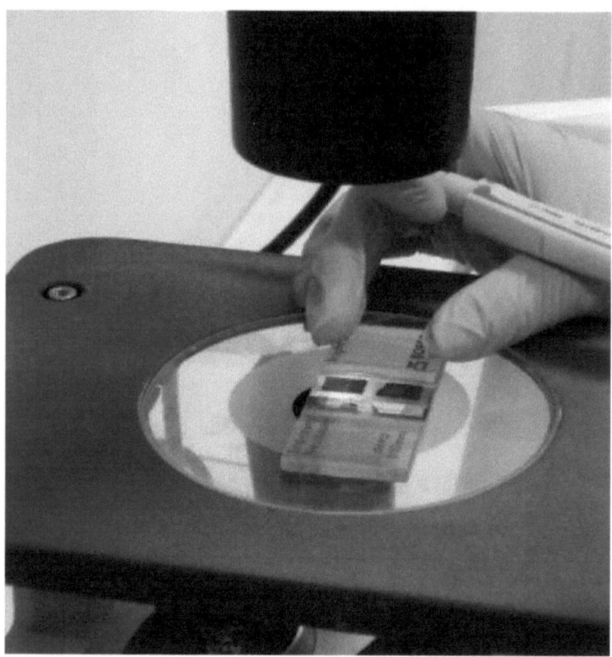

Source: Own authorship.

The total number of cells present in each well at different analysis times was obtained using the following mathematical equation:

Total no. of cells = No. of cells counted X Initial vol. X Dilution X $10^4$ No. of squares used for counting

### 4.2.4 Cytotoxicity evaluation

The cytotoxicity of the endodontic cements used in endodontic filling was evaluated 24, 48 and 72 hours after incubation, and the cell cultures were tested for cell viability using the MTT assay (figure 11). This assay evaluates the ability of metabolically active cells to reduce MTT, converting the yellow salts of tetrazolium (3 - ( 4,5 -dimethylthiazol -2- yl) - 2- 5- diphenyltetrazolium bromide) to formazan crystals, These crystals are purple in color and therefore depend on the ability of the viable cell to cleave the tetrazole ring in MTT by the action of dehydrogenase enzymes present in the active mitochondria, forming formazone crystals.

Figure 11- MTT solution

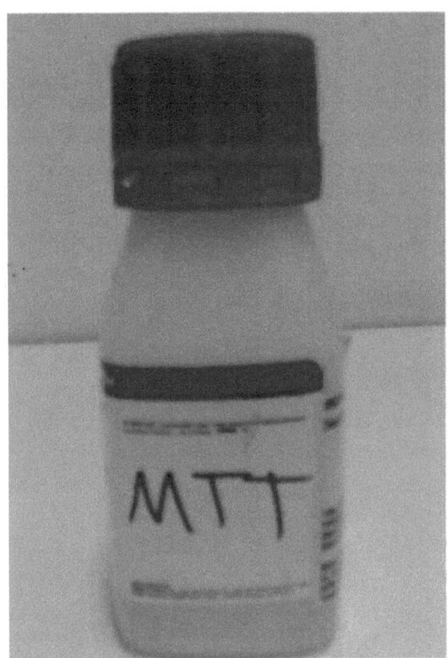

Source: Author

After the crystals had been solubilized, quantification was carried out on an ELX800 multi-plate reader (Epoch biotek instruments, inc.) at 590 nm.

The cytotoxicity test used 110 cells per $mm^2$ in each well of the 96-well thermometer plates (figure 12), incubated with the substances tested for 24, 48 and 72 hours at 37°C. Immediately afterwards, 10 ul of MTT solution (5 mg/mL - SIGMA) diluted in serum-free DMEM culture medium was added to the treated cultures and they were incubated for 4 hours at 37°C. After this incubation period, 100ul of 10% sodium dodecyl sulfate (SDS) solution and 0.01N hydrochloric acid were added and the experiment was maintained for 1 hour at 37°C.

Figure 12- 96 WELL PLATE

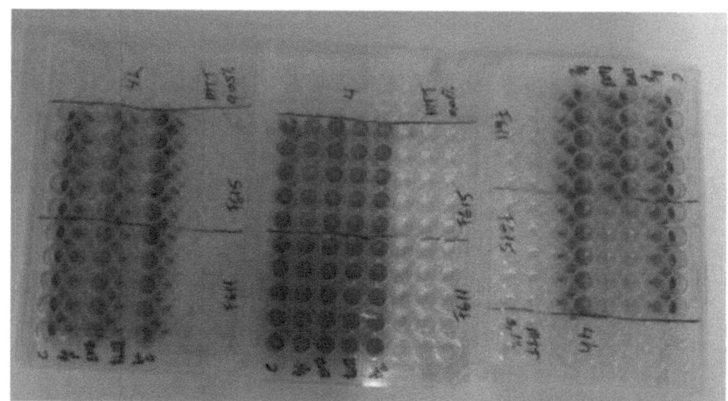

Source: Author

Figure 13- Placing the 96-well plate in the ELX 800 multi-plate reader integrated into the computer, in the Gen 5 program, for the quantification of cell viability using the MTT assay.

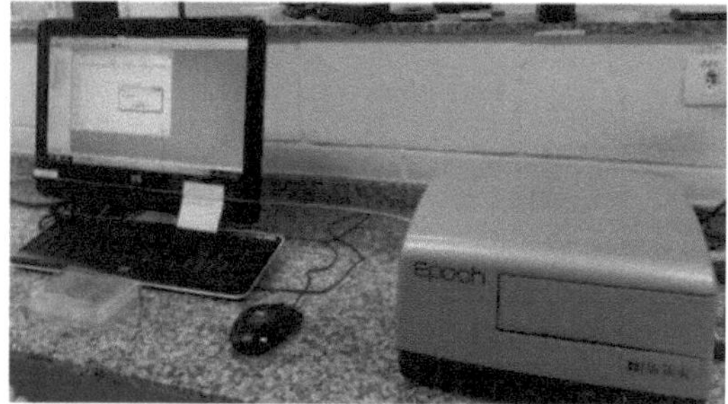

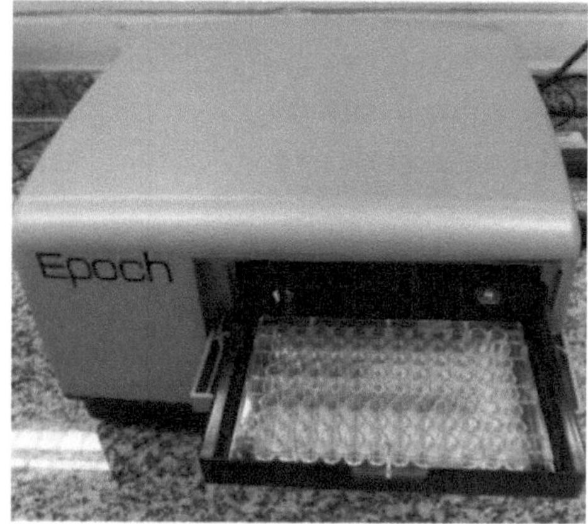

Source: Own authorship.

The optical density of each well will be obtained at 570 nm, making it possible to determine the cytotoxic potential of each substance tested in relation to the control.

## 4.3 Genotoxicity test

The cells were seeded (3 X $10^3$ per cell) on glass slides placed in 35 mm disks on the bottom of the cell culture (figure 14). The cells were incubated for 24 hours at 37°C in a humid atmosphere containing 95% air and 5% carbon dioxide. The culture medium was then replaced with diluted conditioned medium and incubated for 24 hours. After this period, the conditioned medium was discarded and the cells were washed twice with buffered saline. The cells were fixed with 1.5% formaldehyde solution at room temperature for 20 min. The formaldehyde solution was discarded and replaced with cold 100% methanol solution (- 20 °C). The cells were left at room temperature for 20 min. The methanol solution was discarded and the cells were washed three times with PBS. Hoechst solution (Sigma, St Louis, MO, USA) was poured over the cells and incubated for 15 min at room temperature. The glass slides were viewed and photographed using a fluorescence microscope (figure 15). The percentage of micronuclei was determined by the number of cells with micronuclei in 100 cells observed in five specific microscopic fields (at the four extreme points and in the center of the slide) at 400X magnification (figure 16). All experimental groups were tested in triplicate.

Figure 14- Cells seeded on a glass slide.

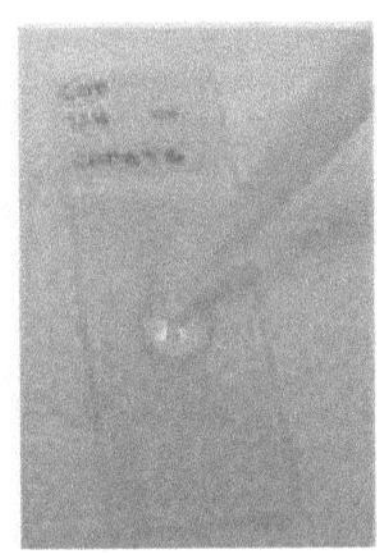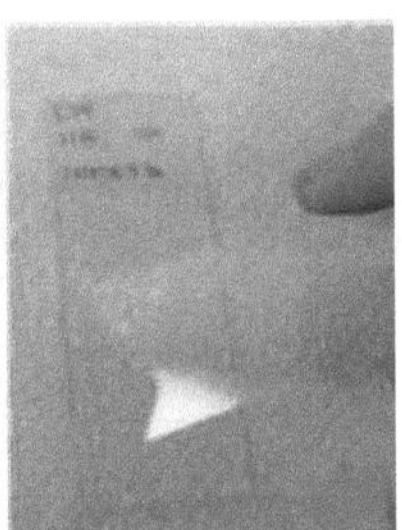

Source: Own authorship.

Figure 15- Fluorescence microscope.

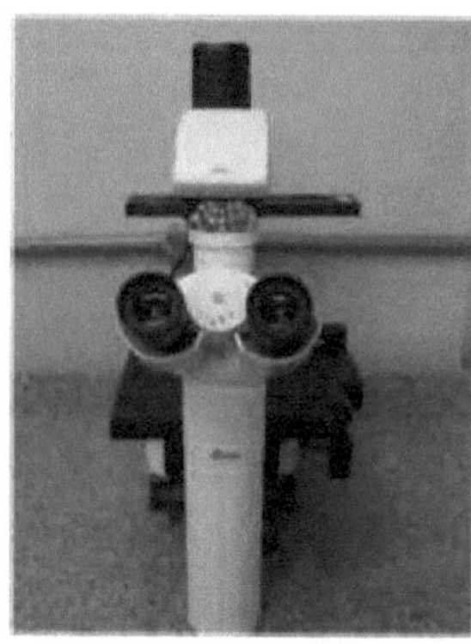

Source: Own authorship.

Figure 16- Formation of micronuclei.

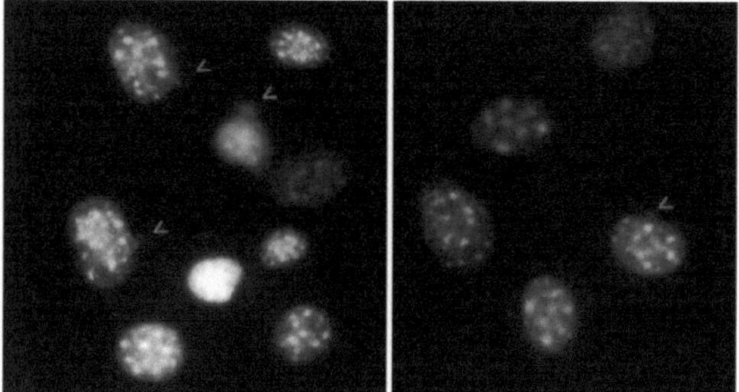

Source: Own authorship.

## 4.4 Analysis of results

The results were analyzed using Biostat 4.0. The Shapiro-Wilk normality test was performed and the sample showed non-normal behavior. A descriptive analysis was carried out and the results were submitted to the Kruskal-Wallis (Dunn) test with a significance level of 5% ($p < 0.05$).

# 5.  RESULTS

Comparing MTA Fillapex, AH Plus and the control group at 24 hours, there was no significant difference in cell proliferation values (p=0.1930). At 48 hours, the highest cell proliferation was found in the control group, with a significant difference compared to MTA (p=0.0058). After 72 hours, the control group showed greater cell proliferation when compared to MTA and AH Plus (p=0.0140) (Table 1 and Graph 1).

Table 1. Medians (MD), interquartile deviations (ID) and Kruskal-Wallis (Dunn) statistical test of cell proliferation of MTA Fillapex, AH Plus and the control group in the same experimental period (number of viable cells x10 ).[4]

| | 24 hours | | | 48 hours | | | 72 hours | | |
|---|---|---|---|---|---|---|---|---|---|
| | MTA | AH P | CT | MTA | AH P | CT | MTA | AH P | CT |
| **MD** | 0.07 | 0.06 | 0.06 | 0.35 | 0.42 | 0.75 | 0.33 | 0.28 | 0.70 |
| **(DI)** | (0.08) | (0.02) | (0.01) | (0.12) | (0.34) | (0.51) | (0.14) | (0.47) | (0.44) |
| | A | A | A | A | AB | B | A | A | B |
| | 0.1930 | | | 0.0058 | | | 0.0140 | | |

Different letters: statistically significant differences

Graph 1. Medians of cell proliferation in MTA Fillapex, AH Plus and the control group over the same experimental period (number of viable cells x10 ).[4]

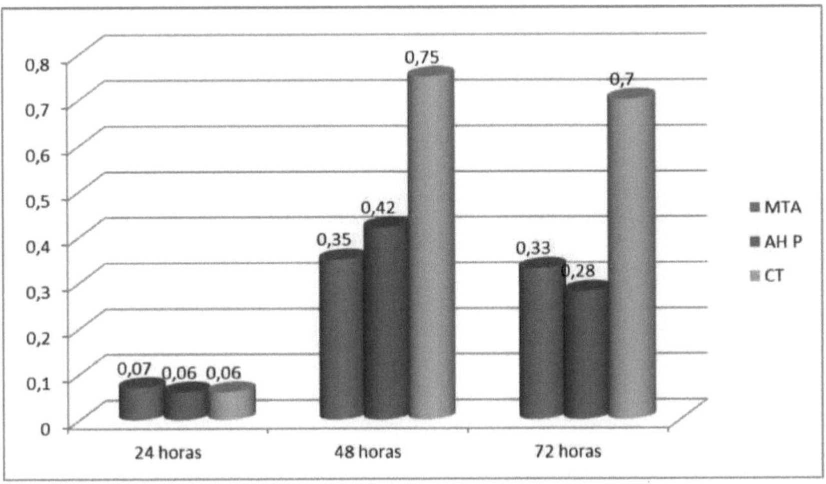


The highest cell viability was observed in the AH Plus cement and the control group in all experimental periods (p≤0.0002, Table 2 and Graph 2).

Table 2. Medians (MD), interquartile deviations (ID) and Kruskal-Wallis statistical test (Dunn) of cell viability of MTA Fillapex, AH Plus and control group (24, 48 and 72 hours).

| | 24 hours | | | 48 hours | | | 72 hours | | |
|---|---|---|---|---|---|---|---|---|---|
| | MTA | AH P | CT | MTA | AH P | CT | MTA | AH P | CT |
| **Viable** | 0.00 (0.02) A | 0.44 (0.15) B | 0.48 (0.13) B | 0.00 (0.00) A | 0.82 (0.40) B | 0.88 (0.44) B | 0.00 (0.00) A | 0.93 (0.60) B | 0.97 (0.54) B |
| **(P)** | 0.0001 | | | 0.0002 | | | 0.0002 | | |
| **Not feasible** | 0.00 (0.04) | 0.00 (0.00) | 0.00 (0.00) | 0.00 (0.00) A | 0.00 (0.00) A | 0.00 (0.00) A | 0.00 (0.00) | 0.00 (0.00) | 0.00 (0.00) |
| **(P)** | 0.3813 | | | 1.0000 | | | 1.0000 | | |

Different capital letters: statistically significant differences

Graph 2. Medians of cell viability of MTA Fillapex, AH Plus and control group (24, 48 and 72 hours)

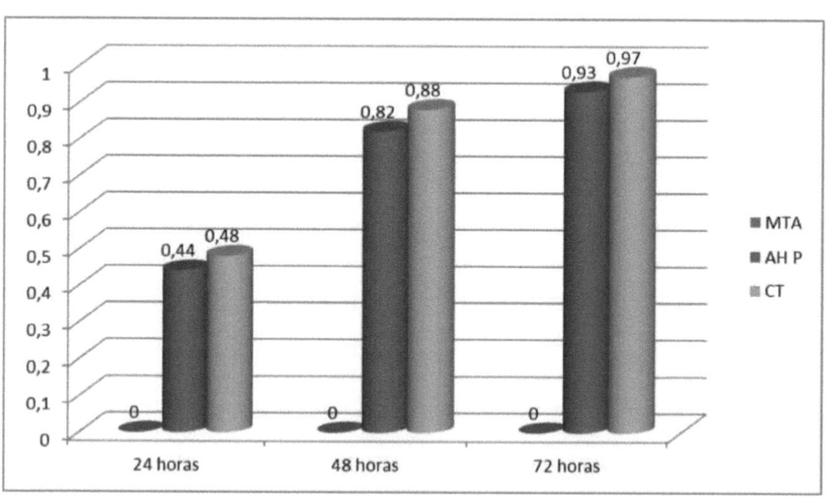


With regard to genotoxicity, the highest value was observed for AH Plus cement after 24 hours, with a significant difference compared to MTA Fillapex and the control group

(p=0.0004) (Table 3 and Graph 3).

Table 3: Medians (MD), interquartile deviations (ID) and Kruskal-Wallis (Dunn) statistical test of the genotoxicity of MTA, AH Plus and the control group over different experimental periods (24, 48 and 72 hours).

| | 24 hours | | | 48 hours | | | 72 hours | | |
|---|---|---|---|---|---|---|---|---|---|
| | MTA | AH P | CT | MTA | AH P | CT | MTA | AH P | CT |
| **MD** (DI) | 0.00 (0.00) A | 2.00 (0.25) B | 0.00 (0.00) A | 0.00 (0.00) A | 1.00 (2.00) A | 0.00 (0.00) A | 0.00 (0.00) A | 1.00 (2.00) A | 0.00 (0.00) A |
| **(P)** | 0.0004 | | | 0.0510 | | | 0.0510 | | |

Different capital letters: statistically significant differences

Graph 3. Medians of the genotoxicity of MTA Fillapex, AH Plus and the control group over different experimental periods (24, 48 and 72 hours).

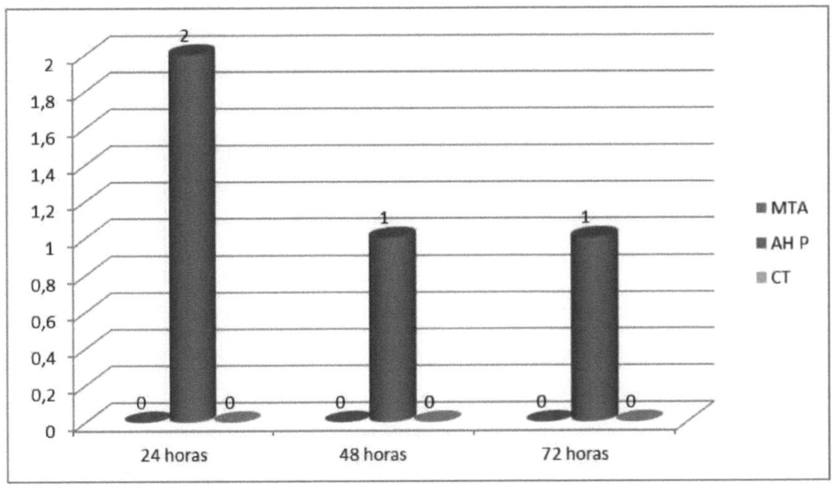

# 6. DISCUSSION

## 6.1 Discussion of methodology

Sealing the canal system using biologically compatible materials continues to be one of the goals of endodontic research. Even with the most modern instrumentation and obturation techniques, in some situations it is difficult to avoid a slight leakage of the obturating material. In this case, the need has arisen for more in-depth studies into biological behavior, without detracting from physical and chemical properties, in an attempt to find a filling cement that will satisfy both the wishes of professionals who work in clinics on a daily basis and researchers in the field (Senne et al., 2009).

To ensure the biocompatibility of endodontic cements, various research methods have been used to evaluate their biological behavior. *In vitro* cytotoxicity tests to analyze the viability or survival of cells are relevant and satisfactory for evaluating the basic biological properties of dental materials, and are less expensive and more reproducible than tests carried out on animals (Camps and About. 2003; Souza et al., 2006).

In this study, human fibroblast culture medium and cell viability assessment techniques such as *Trypan* blue used by Scelza et al. (2001) were used to evaluate cytotoxicity and genotoxicity.

Different types of cells can be used for these types of analysis, and these can come from different types of lineages (Schmalz, 1994; Freshney, 2000). Permanent cell lines are stable, have well-defined biological characteristics and can be obtained from cell culture collections (Schuster et al., 2001). V79 Chinese hamster fibroblasts are widely used because they belong to a previously established cell line and are commercially available. These cells are suitable for analyzing the biological behavior of dental materials due to their stable cellular characteristics (Huang and Chang, 2002).

This study used human fibroblasts, which are the most commonly used cells for establishing permanent lineages, as they are cells that have the capacity to differentiate into multiple cell types and are therefore used in cytotoxicity studies of various compounds (Freshney. 2000).

In several studies, as in this one, the specimens are prepared and placed in a solution in which the materials are able to release their substances forming extracts, with the aim of measuring cytotoxicity and genotoxicity (Schmalz. 1994; Cavalcanti et al., 2005; Camargo et al., 2009). Therefore, the analysis of substances released by the materials during hardening, setting or polymerization can be evaluated (Cavalcanti et al., 2005). After complete hardening, it is still possible that potentially toxic constituents may be released from these filling materials (Huang and Chang, 2002). Therefore, hardening or polymerization of the materials is carried out in an environment with 100% humidity, allowing the study to be more clinically relevant (Cavalcanti et al., 2005).

Eldeniz et al. (2007) reported that the fresher the cement is placed to obtain the extract, the greater the cytotoxicity, and the cements are placed immediately after manipulation. However, it is also important to assess the changes and possible decrease in cytotoxicity over a longer period of time after handling the cements.

In the present study, the cytotoxicity of the endodontic cements used in the filling was evaluated after the specimens had hardened at 24, 48 and 72 hours after incubation, and the cell cultures were tested for cell viability using the MTT assay. The MTT test (3-[4,5-dimethylthiazol-2yl]- 2,5-diphenyltetrazolium bromide) has been used as an *in vitro* cytotoxicity test on cell cultures due to its speed and objectivity. The principle of this test is based on the ability of viable cells to reduce the MTT salt in their mitochondrial metabolism. This reduced salt acquires a purple color, which can be measured in a spectrophotometer using an Elisa reader (Kim et al., 2007). This test was chosen for this study because it offers very accurate results and is sensitive to small changes in cell metabolism.

The most widely used *in vitro* genotoxicity tests are the agarose gel single cell test (or comet test) (Ribeiro et al., 2006) and the micronucleus test (Schweikl and Schmalz. 2000). In this study, the percentage of micronuclei was determined by the number of cells with micronuclei in 100 cells observed in five specific microscopic fields (at the four extreme points and in the center of the slide) at 400X magnification.

## 6.2 Discussion of results

The null hypothesis was rejected because the cements behaved differently.

The substances that make up root canal filling materials can come into contact with the tissues adjacent to the root apex, either through direct contact, in the case of leakage of the filling cement, or due to the diffusion of the degradation products of these substances through numerous connections, such as dentinal tubules, the root canal network, accessory canals, lateral canals, foramina and the apical foramen. Given this fact, the biological properties of these materials are of great importance, since the permanence of a cytotoxic material can result in cellular damage to the tissues adjacent to the root apex. For some authors, only endodontic cements that do not have cytotoxic properties *in vitro* should be indicated in dental practice (Al-Hiyasat., 2010), but if at least these cements provided a minimal cytotoxic action and this action was transient and did not last for long periods, it would already be of great value for their use in endodontic practice.

MTA is a material made up of tricalcium oxide and other oxides such as tricalcium silicate and silicate oxide. Its physical, chemical and biological properties have been tested for some time with good results. Despite these good characteristics, this material does not have the necessary physical properties to be used as an endodontic cement, especially in relation to working and setting time, as well as being difficult to handle (Schwartz et al., 1995; Torabinejad et al., 1995; Roberts et al., 2008; Parirokh &Torabinejad, 2010a, b and c).

MTA cement has good biocompatibility with the adjacent tissues where it is inserted, so it was expected that Fillapex MTA cement, which contains MTA in its formulation, would have a more favorable response when compared to AH Plus cement. However, this hypothesis was not confirmed in this study. MTA Fillapex did not show superior biological behavior to AH Plus. This result is in line with the work carried out by Assman (2013) who mentions that this finding may be related to the presence of a greater quantity of resins in the composition of MTA Fillapex cement than the quantity of MTA.

Knowing the biocompatible characteristics of MTA, Bin et al. (2012) carried out a study comparing the cytotoxicity and genotoxicity of MTA Fillapex cement to AH Plus cement and white MTA in V79 cells. Both AH Plus and MTA Fillapex showed lower rates of cell viability and caused an increase in the formation of micronuclei when compared to the control group. The authors show in this study that MTA Fillapex had the highest cytotoxicity, while white MTA was considered the least toxic and genotoxic in contact with Chinese hamster fibroblast cell culture (V79). A similar result was obtained in the present study, which showed that Fillapex MTA has high cytotoxicity.

Also comparing MTA Fillapex endodontic cement to white MTA cement, Yoshino et al. (2013) evaluated the cytotoxicity of white MTA, MTA Fillapex and Portland cement on human periodontal ligament fibroblasts. MTA Fillapex cement showed the highest cytotoxic levels with reduced cell viability in pure and diluted extracts. They concluded that MTA Fillapex was the material that showed the greatest cytotoxic effect on human periodontal ligament fibroblasts, followed by white MTA and Portland cement.

Following the line of comparative study of MTA Fillapex cement with MTA Couto et al. (2014) carried out a study to analyze the cytotoxicity of MTA Fillapex *in vitro* using gingival fibroblasts. The cells submitted to the MTA-conditioned medium showed a cell growth curve similar to that of the cells in the control group; for the MTA Fillapex group, there was no cell growth and the number of viable cells was significantly lower than in the other groups during the experiment. Thus, the authors concluded that the substances released from MTA Fillapex did not allow cell growth, showing that this MTA-based endodontic cement is highly cytotoxic. The biocompatibility characteristics of MTA may be lost with MTA Fillapex and compromise the success of endodontic treatment.

The cytotoxicity of the two endodontic cements tested in this study showed significant differences. AH Plus resin cement was the least cytotoxic on fibroblast cells, maintaining a good standard of cell viability, showing no significant difference when compared to the control group and in cytotoxicity between all the experimental periods evaluated (24 h, 48 h and 72 h). Silva et al. (2013) tested the cytotoxicity and pH of MTA Fillapex and AH Plus. The authors found that MTA Fillapex was more cytotoxic than AH Plus in all periods, thus agreeing with the results of the present study, which showed that MTA Fillapex was the most cytotoxic in all periods analyzed. When testing the viability of mouse fibroblasts (Balb/c 3T3), keeping cytotoxicity constant over time, AH Plus was moderately cytotoxic initially, slightly cytotoxic after one week and became non-cytotoxic after two weeks.

In contrast, Chang et al. (2014) showed different results to this study, where the aim was to compare the cytotoxicity of four endodontic cements: Sealapex (Sybron Kerr, USA), Apatite Root Sealer (ARS; Dentsply Sankin, Tokyo, Japan), MTA Fillapex (Angellus Industria de Produtos Odontológicos S/A, Londrina, PR, Brazil) and iRoot SP (Innovate BioCreamix Inc, Vancouver, Canada) on human periodontal ligament cells. The MTT results showed that none of the cements evaluated had cytotoxic effects. MTA Fillapex showed favorable growth compared to Sealapex, ARS and iRoot SP for 14 days.

The results of the present study do not agree with Zhou et al. (2015) who carried out a study to evaluate the cytotoxicity of 2 endodontic cements containing calcium silicate. The cements were tested using human gingival fibroblasts. The cements evaluated were EndoSequence BC, MTA Fillapex and the control cement was AH Plus. The authors found that MTA Fillapex was more toxic than AH Plus and BC Sealer at concentrations of 1:2 and 1:8. At concentrations of 1:32 and 1:128, MTA Fillapex was not cytotoxic. The authors concluded that BC Sealer and MTA Fillapex (cements containing calcium silicate in their composition) have different cytotoxicity for human gingival fibroblasts. Perhaps the difference can be explained by the change in concentrations tested.

Silva et al. (2016) carried out a study with similar results to the present study, although with a different methodology, regarding the cytotoxicity of MTA Fillapex cement. The authors evaluated the cytotoxic effects of five endodontic cements (AH Plus,

Endomethasone E, EndoSequence BC, MTA Fillapex and Pulp Canal Sealer EWT) using a three-dimensional (3D) cell culture model. All the cements tested exhibited cytotoxic effects. MTA Fillapex was much more cytotoxic than the other endodontic cements tested.

The genotoxicity of a material is a very relevant aspect and should be considered when choosing an endodontic cement. Contact between a genotoxic cement and periapical tissues can lead to damage to the DNA structure of connective tissue cells, delaying or preventing the repair process (Candeiro et al., 2015).

In relation to genotoxicity, the highest value was found for AH Plus cement in the 24-hour period, with a significant difference compared to MTA Fillapex and the control group. Shweikl & Schmalz (2000) checked the cytotoxicity and genotoxicity of AH Plus cement by means of micronucleus induction in V79 cells. AH Plus was tested immediately after handling and after 24 hours. In this study, no genotoxicity was observed after 24 hours, only immediately after mixing, a result similar to that of the present study. Other authors in previous studies have also observed the positive genotoxicity of AH Plus cement (Schweikl et al., 1998; Huang et al. 2001, 2002; Vandenberg et al., 2007; Camargo et al., 2009 a,b; Soto & Sonnenschein 2010; Bin et al., 2012). In their study, Bin et al. (2012) found severe genotoxicity of AH Plus compared to an MTA-based cement.

It is understood that this study was important in confirming previous results regarding AH Plus and MTA Fillapex, verifying that often a single analysis of the biocompatibility of the cement is not enough, and that a set of tests is necessary to clarify the material's properties in order to assess whether it has the ideal characteristics. According to the results of this study, a material that is cytotoxic is not necessarily genotoxic. Different experimental times should be evaluated, especially for genotoxicity, according to this study.

Studies should be carried out in order to understand the biological behavior of endodontic cements, as well as to continue developing experimental cements that can show more biological effects. As a complement to biological behavior over short periods, it is also important to research the longitudinal effects of different cements in terms of their biocompatibility and resistance to degradation inside the canals. There is also a need to understand the chemical interactions between irrigating solutions, intracanal medications, the dentin substrate and filling materials including gutta-percha, cements and disinfection materials. This information is of fundamental importance in supporting the clinician in choosing the most suitable material for endodontic treatment.

# 7.  CONCLUSION

According to the results of this study, MTA cement

Fillapex showed the greatest cytotoxic potential on human fibroblast cell lines in all experimental periods. With regard to genotoxicity, the highest value was observed for AH Plus cement.

# 8. REFERENCES[i]


Al-Hiyasat AS, Tayyar M, Darmani H. Cytotoxicity evaluation of various resin based root canal sealers. Int Endod J. 2010 Feb;43(2):148-53.

Assman E. Evaluation of the biological behavior of MTA Fillapex cement in rat bone tissue. Dissertation (Master's Degree)-54f. Federal University of Rio Grande do Sul, Porto Alegre, BR, 2013.

Bin CV, Valera MC, Camargo SEA, et al. Cytotoxicity and genotoxicity of root canal sealers based on mineral trioxide aggregate. J Endod. 2012 Feb;38(2); 495-500.

Borges RP, Sousa-Neto MD, Versiani MA et al. Changes in the surface of four calcium silicate-containing endodontic materials and an epoxy-resin-based sealer after a solubility test.Int End J.2012 Mar;38(3): 495-500.

Bouillaguet Wataha JC, Lockwood PE, Galgano C, Golay A, Krejci I. Cytotoxicity and sealing properties of four classes of endodontic sealers evaluated by succinic dehydrogenase activity and confocal laser scanning microscopy Eur J Oral Sci. 2004 Apr;112(2):182-7.

Branstetter J , JA von Fraunhofer. The physical properties of four endodontic sealer cements. J Endod. 1982(8):312-316.

Camargo CH, Camargo SE, Valera MC, Hiller KA, Schmalz G, Schweikl H The induction of cytotoxicity, oxidative stress, and genotoxicity by root canal sealers in mammalian cells. Oral Surgery Oral Medicine Oral Pathology Oral Radiology and Endodontics.Feb (2009a) Oct;108(2):952-60.

Camargo SE, Camargo CH, Hiller KA, Rode SM, Schweikl H, Schmalz G. Cytotoxicity and genotoxicity of pulp capping materials in two cell lines. Int Endod J. (2009b) Mar;42(3):227-37.

Camargo CHR, Oliveira TR, Silva GO, Rabelo SB, Valera MC, Huang TH, Lee H, Kao CT. Evalution of the genotoxicity of zinc oxide eugenol-based, calcium hydroxide-based, and epoxy resin-based root canal sealers by comet assay. Journal Endodontics.2001 May;27(3):744-8.

Camps J. About I. Cytotoxicity testing of endodontic sealers: a new method. J Endod. 2003 Sep;29(9):227-37.


---


[i] According to the 2014 Manual of Normalization for Dissertations and Theses of the Sao Leopoldo Mandic Faculty, based on Vancouver style, and abbreviation of journal titles in accordance with Index Medicus.

Candeiro GT, Correia FC, Duarte MA, et al. Evaluation of radiopacity, pH, release of calcium ions, and flow of a bioceramic root canal sealer J Endod.2012 Oct;(38): 842845.

Candeiro GTM, Moura-Netto C, D'Almeida-Couto RS, Azambuja-Jùnior N, Marques MM, Cai S, Gavini G. Cytotoxicity, genotoxicity and antibacterial effectiveness of a bioceramic endodontic sealer. International Endodontic Journal. 2015 Aug; 11;8(3): 1-7.

Cavalcanti BN, Rode SM, Marques MM. Cytotoxicity of substances leached or dissolved from pulp capping materials. Int Endod J. 2005 Aug;11(8):505-9.

Chang S-W, Lee S-Y, Kang S-K, Kum K-Y, Kim E-C. In Vitro Biocompatibility, Inflammatory Response, and Osteogenic Potential of 4 Root canal Sealers: Sealapex, Sankin Apatite Root Sealer, MTA Fillapex, and iRoot SP Root Canal Sealer. J Endod.2014 Nov; 40:1642-1648.

Cohen S, Hargreaves KM. Pathways to pulp. 9 ed. Sao Paulo: Elsevier Brasil; 2011.

Couto RSD ,Miyagi SPH, Moreira MS, Archilla JR, Marques MM. Cytotoxicity of substances leached from a root canal sealer based on mineral trioxide aggregate Clin Lab Res Den 2014 Jun;20(3):145-51.

Eldeniz AU, Mustafa K, Orstavik D, Dahl JE. Cytotoxicity of new resin-calcium hydroxide- and silicone-based root canal sealers on fibroblasts derived from human gingiva and L929 cell lines. Int Endod J. 2007 Feb;(2):126-35.

Freshney RI. Culture of animal Cell: a manual of basic technique. 4ed. Indianapolis: Wiley Liss;2000.

Gomes-Filho JE, Watanabe C, Lodi CS et al. Effect of MTA-based sealer on the healing of periapical lesions. J Appl Oral Sci. 2013;21(3):235-242,.

Huang FM, Hsieh YS, Tai KW, Chou MY, Chang YC. Induction of c-fos and c-jun protooncogenes expression by formaldehyde-releasing and epoxy resin-based rootcanal sealers in human osteoblastics cells. Journal of Biomedical Material Research. 2002;59:460-5.

Huang FM, Yai KW, Chou MY, Chang YC. Cytotoxicity of resin-zinc oxide-eugenol and calcium hydroxide-based root canal sealers on human periodontal ligament permanent V79 cells. Int Endod J. 2002 Feb;35(2):153-8.

Karapinar-Kazandag M, Bayrak OF, Yalvac ME, Ersev H, Tanalp J, Sahin F, et al. Cytotoxicity of 5 endodontic sealers on L929 cell line and human dental pulp cells. Int Endod J. 2011 Feb;44(7):626-34.

Kim E, Jeon IS, Kim JW, Kim J, Jung HS, Lee SJ. An MTT-based method for quantification of periodontal ligament cell viability. Oral Dis.2007 Sep;13(5):495-9.

Lee JK, Kim DB, Kim JI, Kim PY. In vitro cytotoxicity tests on cultured human skin fibroblasts to pedict skin irritation potential of surfactants. Toxicol Vitr. 2000 Aug; 14(4):345-9.

Leonardo MR, da Silva LA, Almeida WA, Utrilla LS. Tissue response to na epoxy resin-based root canal sealer. Endod Dent Trumatol, 1999;15:28-32.

Leonardo MR, Flores DS, de Paula ESFW, de Toledo Leonardo R, da Silva LA. A comparison study of periapical repair in dogs' teeth using RoekoSeal and AH plus root canal sealers: a histopathological evaluation. J Endod. 2008 Jul;34(7):822-5.

Lodiene G, Morisbak E, Bruzell E, Orstavik D. Toxicity evaluation of root canal sealers in vitro. Int Endod J. 2008 Jan;41(1):72-7.

Lopes HP, Siqueira Jr JF, Endodontics: biology and technique / Hélio Pereira Lopes, José Freitas Siqueira Jr.- 3.ed.- Rio de Janeiro: Guanabara Koogan, 2010. p. 613-639.

Loushine BA, Bryan TE, Looney SW, et al. Setting properties and cytotoxicity evaluation of a premixed bioceramic root canal sealer. J Endod .2011;37:673-677.

Marques NCT, et al. Rat Subcutaneous Tissue Response to MTA Fillapex and Portland Cement. Braz Dental J, Riberao Preto. 2013;24(1):10-14,.

Miletic I, Anic I, Karlovic Z, Mars"an T, Pezelj-Ribaric S, Osmak M. Cytotoxic effect of four root filling materials. Endodontics and Dental Traumatology. 2003 Dec; 16(6): 287-90.

Miletic I, Devcic N, Anic I, Borcic J, Karlovic Z, Osmak M. The cytotoxicity of RoekoSeal and AH Plus compared during different setting periods. J Endod. 2005 Apr;31(4):307-9.

Nagas E, Uyanik O, Eymirili A, et al. Dentin moisture conditions affect the adhesion of root canal sealers. J Endod. 2012;38:240-244.

Nguyen TN. Filling root canal systems. In: . Cohen S, Burns, editor RC Pulp Pathways. 4th ed. St Louis, MO: Mosby, 1987, p. 183-194.

Parirokh M, Torabinejad M. Mineral trioxide aggregate: a comprehensive literature review-part I: chemical, physical, and antibacterial properties. J Endod. 2010;36:16- 27.

Parirokh M, Torabinejad M. Mineral trioxide aggregate: a comprehensive literature review-part III: clinical applications, drawbacks, and mechanism of action. J Endod. 2010;36:400-13.

Ray HA, Trope M. Periapical status of endodontically treated teeth in relation to the technical quality of the root filling and the coronal restoration. Endod Int J. 1995;12- 18.

Ribeiro DA, Marques ME, Salvadori DM. Lack of genotoxicity foformocresol, paramonochlorophenol and calcium hydroxide on mammalian cells by comet assay. J Endod. 2004 Aug;30(8):593-6.

Ribeiro DA, Sugui MM, Matsumoto MA, Duarte MA, Marques ME, Salvadori DM. Genotoxicity and cytotoxicity of mineral trioxide aggregate and regular and white Portland cements on Chinese hamster ovary (CHO) cells in vitro. Oral Surg Oral Med Oral Pathol Oral Radiol Endod. 2006 Feb;101(2):258-61.

Roberts HW, Toth JM, Berzins DW, Charlton DG. Mineral trioxide aggregate material use in endodontic treatment: a review of the literature. Dent Mat. 2008;24:149-64.

Santos J, Tjaderhane L, Ferraz C, et al Long-term sealing ability of resin- based root canal fillings. Endod Int J. 2010;43:455-460.

Scarparo RK, Grecca FS, Fachin EVF. Analysis of tissue reactions to methacrylate resin-based, epoxy resin-based, and zinc oxide-eugenol endodontic sealers. J Endod. 2009;35:229-232.

Scarparo RK, Fachin EVF, Grecca FS. Methodologies for the preliminary evaluation of the biocompatibility of endodontic materials in connective tissue: a literature review. Ver Fac Odontol Porto Alegre. 2010;50:32-35.

Scelza MF, Daniel RL, Santos EM, Jaeger MM. Cytotoxicity effects of 10% citric acid and EDTA-T used as root canal irrigants: an in vitro analysis. J Endod. 2001;27(12):741-43.

Schilder H. Filling root canals in three dimensions. Dent Clin North Am. 1967;11: 723-744.

Schmalz G. Use of cell cultures for toxicity testing of dental materials advantages and limitations.J Dent. 1994;22 Suppl2:S6-11.

Schuster U, Schmalz G, Thonemann B, Mendel N, Metzl C. Cytotoxicity testing with three-dimensional cultures of transfected pulp-derived cells. J Endod. 2001 Apr;27(4):259-65.

Schwartz R, Mauger M, Clement D, Walker WA. Mineral trioxide aggregate: a new material for endodontics. J Am Dent Assoc, 1999;130:967-975.

Schweikl H, Schmalz G. The induction of micronuclei in V79 cells by the root canal filling material AH Plus. Biomaterials. 2000 May;21(9):939-44.

Senne MI, Lemos N, Fidel RAS. Evaluation of the cytotoxicity of three root canal sealers used in obturation of radicular canals system. RSBO. 2009;6(1):71-76.

Silva EJ, Rosa TP, Herrera DR, et al. Evaluation of cytotoxicity and physicochemical properties of calcium silicate-based endodontic sealer MTA Fillapex. J Endod. 2013;39:274-7.

Silva EJ, Carvalho NK, Ronconi CT, De Deus G, Zuolo ML, Zaia AA. Cytotoxicity Profile of Endodontic Sealers Provided by 3D Cell Culture Experiment. Braz Dent J. 2016;27:1-6.

Siqueira JF Jr, Favieri A, Gahyva SM et al. Antimicrobial activity and flow rate of newer and stabilized root canal sealers. J Endod. 2000:26:274-7.

Soares IJ, Goldberg F. Endodontia - Tècnica e Fundamentos. 2.ed. Porto Alegre: Artmed; 2011. p. 221-249.

Soto AM, Sonnenschein C. Environmental causes of cancer: endocrine disruptors as carcinogens. Nature Reviews Endocrinology. 2010;6:363-70.

Souza NJA, Justo GZ, Oliveira CR, Haun M, Bincoletto C. Cytotoxicity of materials used in perforation repair tested using the V79 fibroblast cell line and the granulocyte-macrophage progenitor cells. Int Endod J. 2006;39(1):40-7.

Taintor JF, Ross PN. Opinions and practices of American Endodontic Diplomates. J Dent. 1978;44:321-325.

Torabinejad M, Hong CU, Pit Ford TR, Kettering JD. Cytotoxicity of four root end filling materials. J Endod. 1995;21:489-492.

Torabinejad M, Parirokh M. Mineral trioxide aggregate: a comprehensive literature review - part II: leakage and biocompatibility investigations. J Endod. 2010;36:190- 202.

Torabinejad M, Smith PW, Kettering JD, Pitt Ford TR. Comparative investigation of marginal adaptation of mineral trioxide aggregate and other commonly used root-end filling materials. J Endod. 1995;21:295-9.

Vandenberg LN, Hauser R, Marcus M, Olea N, Welshons WV (2007) Human exposure to bisphenol A (BPA). Reproductive Toxicology. 2007;24:139-77.

Versiani MA, Carvalho-Junior JR, Padilha MI, Lacey S, Pascon EA, Sousa-Neto MD.

Walton RE, Torabinejad M. Principles and Practices in Endodontics. 3ed. Philadelphia: Saunders; 2002.

Yoshino P, Nishiyama CK, Modena KCS, Santos CF, Sipert CR. *In Vitro* cytotoxicity of white MTA, MTA Fillapex and Portland cement on human periodontal ligament fibroblasts.

Braz Dent J. 2013;24(2):111-116.

Zhang H, Shen Y, Ruse ND, Haapasalo M,. Antibacterial activity of endodontic sealers by modified direct contact test against Enterococcus faecalis. J Endod. 2009;35:1051-1055.

Zhou H, Du T, Shen Y, Wang Z, Zheng Y, Haapasalo M. In Vitro Cytotoxicity of Calcium Silicate-containing Endodontic Sealers. J Endod. 2015;41:56-61.

# ANNEX A: OPINION OF THE ETHICS COMMITTEE

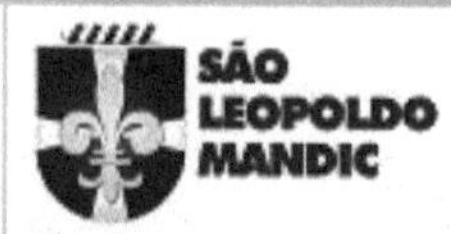


FACULDADE SÃO LEOPOLDO
MANDIC

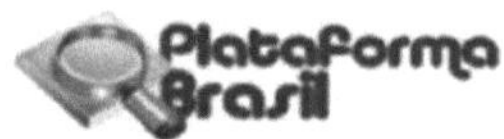


## EXECUTIVE OPINION OF THE CEP

RESEARCH PROJECT DATA

Research Title: Analysis of cytotoxicity, genotoxicity and o pH of endodontic cements MTA Fillapex and AH plus in human fibroblasts

Researcher: CAMiLA DE PAIVA MACEDO

Thematic Area:

Version: 1

CAAE: 63345516.0.0000.5374

Proponent Institution: Cent' o de Pôs-Graduaçâo Sâo Leopoldo MandicZFaculty of Main Sponsor: Own Funding

OPINION DATA

Opinion Number: 1.921.764

Project presentation:

An experimental in vitro study will be carried out using gingival fibroblast cells from the Cell Bank of the Sao Leopoldo Mandic Institute and Research Center (Campinas, Sao Paulo), which have already been approved by the Ethics Committee of this institution (protocol n. 2012/0308). Human fibroblast cell lines obtained from three different patients and stored in the Cell Bank will be used in order to consider the phenotypic and genotypic variations of the different cells in relation to a biomaterial. This in vitro study aims to

The aim is to evaluate the cytotoxic, genotoxic and pH potential of MTA fillapex endodontic cement (Angelus, Londrina, PR, Brazil) compared to AH plus cement (Dentsply$_1$ Konstanz, Germany). In addition,$_1$ will evaluate the behavior of fibroblast cells after 24h, 48h and 72h, the proliferation and viability of gingival fibroblasts, using Trypan blue and MTT vital dye, respectively. The data will be tabulated and submitted to an appropriate statistical test, using a 5% significance level.

Research Objective:

The aim of this study was to evaluate the cytotoxic, genotoxic and pH potential of MTA Fillapex endodontic cement (Angelus, Londrina$_1$ PR$_1$ Brasil) by comparing it with o cement

**Endereço:** Rua José Rocha Junqueira Nº13
**Bairro:** Swift        **CEP:** 13.045-755
**UF:** SP    **Municipio:** CAMPINAS
**Telefone:** (19)3518-3601    **Fax:** (19)3211-3600    **E-mail:** cep@slmandic.edu.br

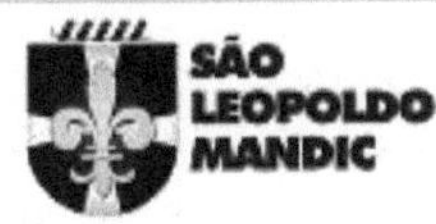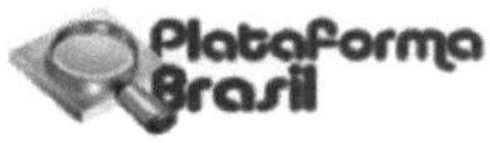

# FACULDADE SÃO LEOPOLDO MANDIC



endodontic AH Plus (Dentsply, Konstanz, Germany).

Assessment of risks and benefits:

Adequately described.

Comments and Considerations on the Research:

Adequate for what it sets out to investigate.

Consideration of mandatory terms of presentation:

Satisfactorily presented.

Conclusions or Pendencies and List of Inadequacies:

No pending issues.

Final considerations at the discretion of the CEP:

The researcher should be aware that the research project approved by this CEP refers to the protocol SUBMITTED for evaluation, and the CEP is exempt from co-responsibility for research already carried out. Therefore, in accordance with CNS Resolution 466/12, the researcher is responsible for "developing the project as outlined", and if there are any changes to this project, this CEP must be notified in an amendment via Piataforma Brasil, for a new assessment.

This opinion has been drawn up on the basis of the documents listed below:

| Document Type | Archive | Post | Author | Situation |
|---|---|---|---|---|
| Basic Project Information | PB_BASIC_INFORMATION ROJECT 845946.pdf | 21/12/2016 13:16:14 | | Accepted |
| Biological Material Handling Declaration / Biorepository / Biobank | 987654321 .pdf | 20/12/2016 08:21:16 | CAMILA DE PAIVA MACEDO | Accepted |
| Cover Sheet | 20161219110055680.pdf | 20/12/2016 08:20:54 | CAMILA DE PAIVA MACEDO | Accepted |
| ICF / Terms of Assent / Justification for Absence | 1234567.doex | 19/12/2016 10:53:18 | CAMILA DE PAIVA MACEDO | Accepted |
| Statement of Institution and Infrastructure | 7654321.pdf | 19/12/2016 10:50:18 | CAMILA DE PAIVA MACEDO | Accepted |
| Detailed Design | 1234567.doc | 19/12/2016 | CAMILA DE PAIVA | Accepted |

**Endereço:** Rua José Rocha Junqueira Nº13
**Bairro:** Swift                         **CEP:** 13.045-755
**UF:** SP        **Município:** CAMPINAS
**Telefone:** (19)3518-3601      **Fax:** (19)3211-3600      **E-mail:** cep@slmandic.edu.br

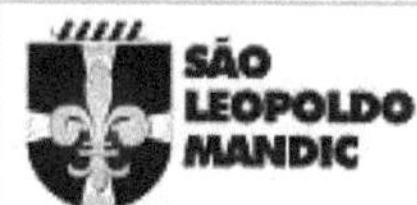
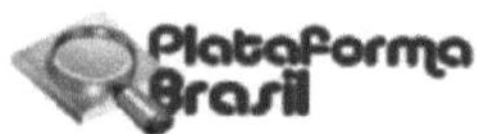

# FACULDADE SÃO LEOPOLDO MANDIC



| / Brochura Investigador | 1234567.doc | | 10:46:00 | MACEDO | Aceito |
| --- | --- | --- | --- | --- | --- |

**Situação do Parecer:**
Aprovado

**Necessita Apreciação da CONEP:**
Não

CAMPINAS, 15 de Fevereiro de 2017

**Assinado por:**
**Fabiana Mantovani Gomes França**
**(Coordenador)**

# ANNEX B. AUTHORIZATION TO USE THE LABORATORY

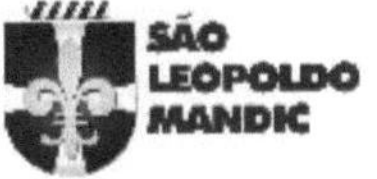


Campinas, 15 de dezembro de 2016.

## DECLARATION

I hereby declare that the human gingival ftbroblast cells are in the Cell Bank of the Cell Culture Laboratory of the Sâo Leopoldo Mandic Institute and Research Center for use in research, and that their isolation has already been approved by this Committee in a previous project {protocol 2012/D30β). Furthermore, I am aware of and authorize its use by the student Camila de **Paiva** Macedo, in order to proceed with her master's project.

Conditionally

Profa. Dra. Elizabeth Ferreira Martinez


SLMandic – R. José Rocha Junqueira, 13 – Campinas - SP
CEP: 13045-755 - Fone: (019) 3211-3625
E-Mail: efmartinez@ig.com.br

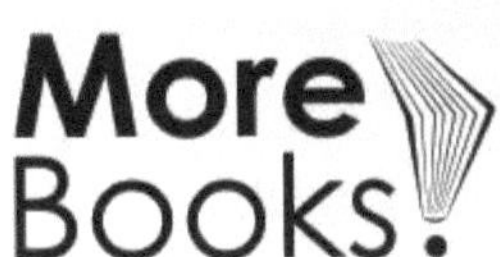


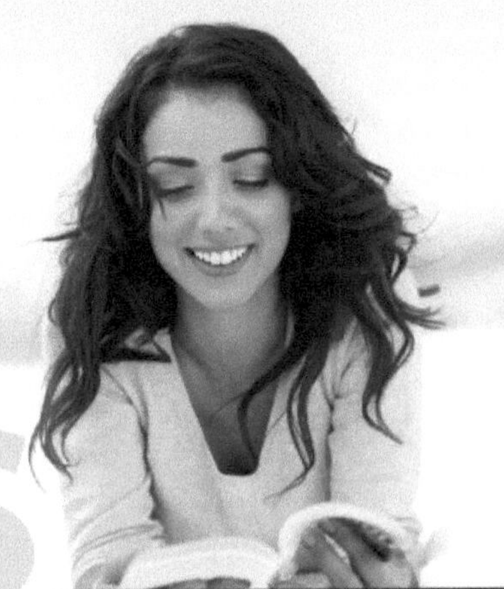



# I want morebooks!

Buy your books fast and straightforward online - at one of world's fastest growing online book stores! Environmentally sound due to Print-on-Demand technologies.

Buy your books online at
## www.morebooks.shop

Kaufen Sie Ihre Bücher schnell und unkompliziert online – auf einer der am schnellsten wachsenden Buchhandelsplattformen weltweit! Dank Print-On-Demand umwelt- und ressourcenschonend produzi ert.

Bücher schneller online kaufen
## www.morebooks.shop

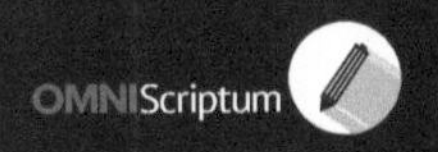

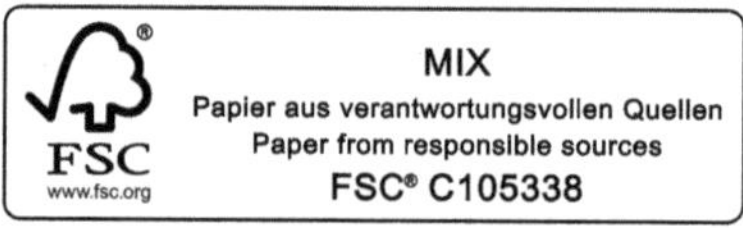

Printed by Books on Demand GmbH, Norderstedt / Germany